Professional Development

Edited by
Kathleen Kendall-Tackett, PhD, IBCLC, FAPA
& Scott Sherwood, BS

All royalties go to the
U.S. Lactation Consultant Association.

Praeclarus Press, LLC
©2015. United States Lactation Consultant Association

Praeclarus Press, LLC

2504 Sweetgum Lane

Amarillo, Texas 79124 USA

806-367-9950

www.PraeclarusPress.com

DISCLAIMER

The information contained in this publication is advisory only and is not intended to replace sound clinical judgment or individualized patient care. The author disclaims all warranties, whether expressed or implied, including any warranty as the quality, accuracy, safety, or suitability of this information for any particular purpose.

ISBN: 978-1-939807-33-5

Cover Design: Ken Tackett

Acquisition & Development: Kathleen Kendall-Tackett & Scott Sherwood

Copy Editing: Kathleen Kendall-Tackett & Chris Tackett

Layout & Design: Nelly Murariu

Operations: Scott Sherwood

Contents

USLCA

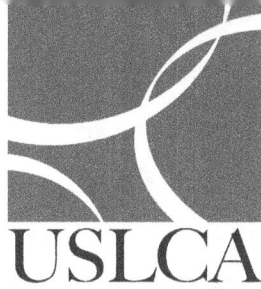

From Volunteer to Professional
The Journey to Becoming Lactation Consultants

Vicki Tapia, BA, IBCLC, RLC[1]
Diane Powers, BA, IBCLC, RLC[2]

Keywords: Volunteer, breastfeeding support, IBCLC

Many of the founders of the field of human lactation started as volunteers. Eventually, this army of volunteers wanted professional recognition for their clinical skills and knowledge about breastfeeding. Many who currently aspire to become IBCLCs volunteer to help new mothers while acquiring the hours and courses they need to sit for the exam. This article chronicles the journeys of two IBCLCs who started down the volunteer-to-professional path in the early days of our field.

1   victorialee37@gmail.com
2   dpowers@billingsclinic.org

In 1987, the profession of lactation consulting was in its infancy. ILCA and IBCLE had gained visibility only two years prior. We came together sharing the common belief that we could make a difference in the lives of breastfeeding women, one mother at a time. The time had arrived to turn a volunteer position as La Leche League Leaders into a profession!

Our vision became the first step of a long journey. As with many new endeavors into uncharted territory, the first steps are often missteps. Laying the groundwork, we decided to create a brochure describing our services. Many hours and painstaking edits later, we beheld 500 brochures, printed at a local shop, which we mailed to each new mother listed in the birth announcements in our local newspaper. To our dismay, no one responded, and we learned the birth announcements were listed several days after the baby's actual birth date. We needed a method of reaching mothers during pregnancy. In 1987, in our community of 90,000, there were eight obstetricians and nine pediatricians. Only one obstetrician and one pediatrician were supportive of our vision and referred mothers to our service. The obstetrician also agreed to include our brochure in the information packet given to all pregnant patients.

Our next step was to educate the medical community regarding our business, and also, the strong need for our service. *Breastfeeding Update,* a one-page bi-monthly newsletter addressing common problems and issues concerning breastfeeding, was printed and mailed to all obstetricians, pediatricians, family medicine physicians, birthing instructors, and the hospital maternity nurse manager. We contacted nurses from the different pediatric and OB clinics, as well as the hospital maternity nurses, scheduling a luncheon at each office for which we furnished a gourmet lunch they enjoyed while we explained our services.

In addition, when we received a referral from a physician, we made it our practice to send this physician a concise follow-up letter. We contacted both pediatric and obstetric offices, asking to be scheduled into their doctor's meeting as speakers to outline our services.

Looking back, we were fairly fearless when facing a group of physicians, most of whom were polite, but uninterested in our proposal of a lactation consulting service.

Our 45-minute breastfeeding overview at childbirth classes provided by the obstetricians gave us the opportunity to share information and hand out our brochures to mothers before they delivered. This became a growing source of referrals. Hospital visits, home visits, and counseling calls continued to trickle in, and it became apparent that laying the groundwork took a lot of time and energy with few immediate results.

Word-of-mouth by satisfied clients was our best source of new business. The hospital could no longer ignore us. The letters of complaint from our unsatisfied customers, who were frustrated by the inconsistent lactation information, were the catalysts that irritated hospital administration to the point of demanding that we have staff privileges before making any more visits to new mothers in the hospital.

This new roadblock was actually an important step. If we could secure hospital privileges, this would give us credibility with the medical community. The next question was how to accomplish this. In part, because our degrees were in education, and no one without a medical degree had ever been granted privileges to this hospital, it was new to them. If the powers-that-be thought this obstacle would discourage us, they were simply unaware at how tenacious we were. We forged ahead, inquiring about the application process, and were given a stack of paperwork to complete. It was necessary to find a sponsoring physician, plus liability insurance of $1,000,000.

A meeting was scheduled between the obstetrics department chair and ourselves. Attired in suits, with briefcases in hand, we confidently marketed our knowledge and skills. The meeting was a success, which meant we had found our sponsor. We completed the application for hospital privileges in March 1989. Thus began the waiting process as the applications were processed through cumbersome and tedious hospital departments and committees. We also began searching for a source of liability insurance. None of the insurance companies had ever heard of lactation consultants. We eventually found a company that was willing to insure us under an umbrella policy similar to one for nurses. After we sent them our money, we could not shake the feeling that they laughed all the way to the bank.

In the meantime, we continued sporadic hospital and home visits, although the atmosphere on the maternity floor often felt strained. We continued to publish our *Breastfeeding Update*, speak at childbirth classes, and make infrequent visits to new mothers, while waiting to hear about our applications for hospital privileges.

Our journey took a new turn in 1989, with an invitation that became our first big break. We were invited to give away long in-service for nurses, nursing students, and dietitians in a community two hours away. The evaluations were very positive and we were ecstatic. The euphoria lasted one week, until the nurse manager at our hospital mentioned she heard we had put on a nice little LLL-style in-service, and she went on to attack our professionalism.

Taking careful notes during the conversation, we were able to respond to her comments with 33 evaluations, of which over 90% gave us an *excellent* overall rating, along with a favorable recommendation from the conference coordinator. Copies of this letter went to appropriate hospital chairpersons and directors. The nurse manager's cryptic apology was followed coincidentally by her resignation the following month.

By July of 1989, we had reached a crossroad. The pressure and disappointment of not hearing any news about hospital privileges, the dollars needed to reprint our brochures, combined with an income level as low as our morale, brought us to the brink of drafting a letter to thank our supporters and resign ourselves to a different vision. Anything seemed better than the bleak outlook of more battles with the established medical community.

August arrived. Almost simultaneously, our hospital privileges were approved (we became the only non-medically degreed people to have privileges), and the Children's Clinic contracted with us to visit all their breastfeeding mothers each day of their hospital stay. We each worked three mornings a week. We had arrived!

In September 1989, two years and five months after embarking on our odyssey, we began our new journey as lactation consultants visiting new mothers in the hospital. We also were given space by a local obstetrician to offer bi-monthly prenatal breastfeeding classes for $5/couple, in exchange for continuing to offer the free introductory informational talks at childbirth classes a couple times per month. In the Fall of 1990, after months of our suggestions to this effect, the Children's Clinic added clinic visits to our job description. We then began to see mothers at the baby's first clinic visit four days after hospital discharge.

In 1994, we sat for the IBCLE exam, thus gaining our certification as IBCLC. More than 20,000 mother/baby dyads later, we have not lost sight of our journey to make a difference, one mother at a time. However, we have also broadened our journey to include speaking professionally at conferences, both nationally and internationally, as well as writing for the *Journal of Human Lactation* (JHL), and other publications.

We continue to make daily rounds at both hospitals, as well as see new mothers and babies in our respective clinics post discharge. There is no charge to the mother for our service. From the beginning, our support and service has been quietly underwritten by the physicians with whom we work. These physicians are the wind beneath our wings, allowing us to provide expertise and encouragement to mothers from all walks of life in our community.

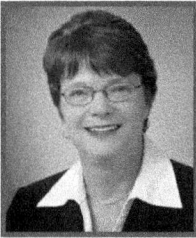

Diane Powers, BA, IBCLC, RLC, is a lactation consultant and former La Leche League leader. For the past 23 years, she has worked with approximately 700 new mother/baby pairs per year, both in-patient and outpatient. She has completed two research projects and had numerous articles published. She lectures nationally and internationally.

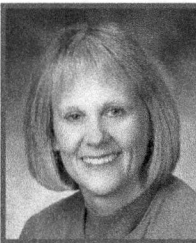

Vicki Bodley Tapia, B.S., IBCLC, RLC, is a former La Leche League Leader, and has been in private practice as a lactation consultant since 1987, published numerous articles, and lectures both nationally and internationally.She is the author of *Somebody Stole My Iron: A Family Memoir of Dementia* from Praeclarus Press.

USLCA

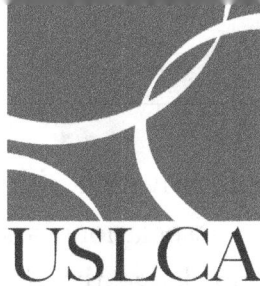

Improving the Bottom-Line

Financial Justification for the Hospital-Based Lactation Consultant Role

Shannon Francis-Clegg, BSN, MBA, IBCLC, RLC[4]
Deanne T. Francis, BSN, IBCLC, RLC, LCCE[5]

Intermountain Healthcare Lactation Standardization Project (2007)[6]

Keywords: lactation care, breastfeeding support, lactation-failure readmissions, optimal lactation care

Intermountain Healthcare's Lactation Standard Team conducted a year-long in-depth study to evaluate their current lactation services for staffing, patient satisfaction, patient and staff education, reimbursement patterns, cost of care and lactation-failure readmissions. The attempt was to evaluate and then standardize the lactation services within their 23-hospital system, and create staffing recommendations to support optimal lactation care and support. This article represents a brief summary of recommendations based on this study. Individual portions of the project with detailed process and final results/data will be submitted for future publication.

4   Intermountain Healthcare, shannon.clegg@imail.org
5   Intermountain Healthcare
6   Team Members: Project Lead: Shannon Clegg BSN, MBA, IBCLC. Project Team Members: Janeva Babbel, RN, IBCLC; Sue Bedard, RNC, MSN, IBCLC; Margo Christensen, RN, IBCLC; Cheryl DeMille, RN, BSN, IBCLC; Diana Dennis, BSN, IBCLC; Deanne Francis, RNC, IBCLC, LCCE; Lynn Gardner,RN, BA, IBCLC; Erick Henry, MPH; Terese Larkin,RN, BSN, IBCLC; Ellen Lechtenberg, RD, CSP, IBCLC; Kayleen Ragozzine, RNC, BSN, IBCLC; Janis Sumsion,RN, IBCLC.

Most government, private health care organizations, national professional associations, and a majority of the general public, acknowledge that breastfeeding is the normal, standard, and optimal way to feed the human infant (American Academy of Pediatrics, 2005; American Academy of Family Physicians, 2010; American College of Obstetricians & Gynecologists, 2007; Association of Women's Health, Obstetric & Neonatal Nurses, 2010; Centers for Disease Control and Prevention, 2010). However, in the current health care environment, some organizations are cutting lactation services in an attempt to improve their financial bottom-line.

This is being done despite the fact that well-documented data shows that sub-optimal U.S. breastfeeding rates are linked to excess costs and infant deaths. A recent study by Bartick and Reinhold (2010) shows that if 90% of U.S. families could comply with medical recommendations to breastfeed exclusively for 6 months, potential U.S. savings of $13 billion per year, and prevention of an excess of 911 deaths could be realized. Nearly all of these benefits would be realized in infants ($10.5 billion and 741 deaths at 80% compliance). Yet, most states are well below the *Healthy People* 2010 and 2020 national breastfeeding objectives. [Click here for CDC State Report Cards: http://www.cdc.gov/breastfeeding/pdf/2014breastfeedingreportcard.pdf]

In 2010, the Joint Commission issued a new Perinatal Core Measure Set (an evidence-based tool to afford accredited hospitals the opportunity to use a standardized approach for assessing quality in perinatal care,) specifically to improve exclusive breast-milk feeding in the hospital.

Core Measure Sets must be selected in their entirety, so hospitals that wish to include the Perinatal Core Measures as part of their ORYX[4] reporting need to include the breastfeeding measure.

The most current data on exclusive breast-milk feeding rates indicate that many hospitals likely will face a substantial challenge in showing improvement in this measure. It will be critical for hospitals to initiate or improve services, support, and programs that will help achieve this measure.

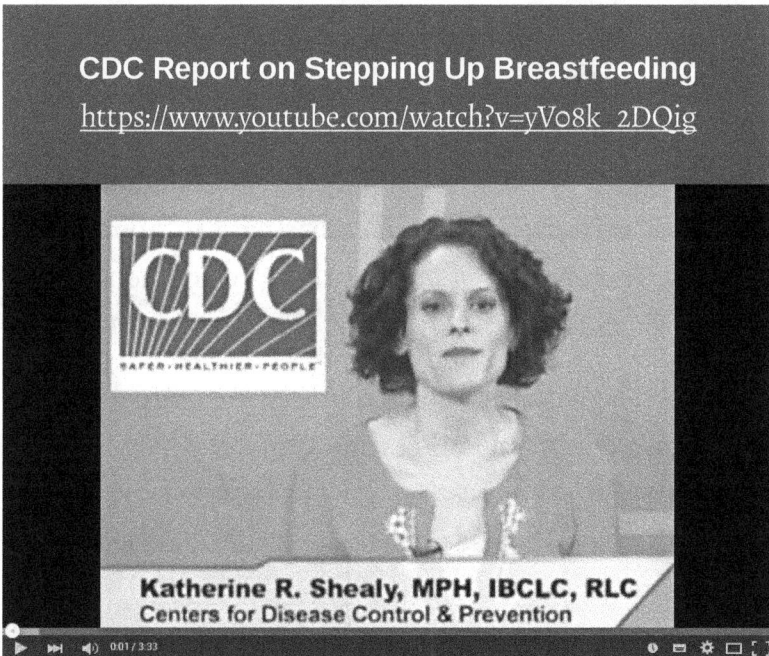

CDC Report on Stepping Up Breastfeeding
https://www.youtube.com/watch?v=yVo8k_2DQig

Katherine R. Shealy, MPH, IBCLC, RLC
Centers for Disease Control & Prevention

---

4   ORYX: A quality-improvement initiative that reflects the increasing use and importance of performance measures in U.S. medical practice.

Study of the Quality and Consistency of Lactation Care at Intermountain HealthCare

In an attempt to improve the quality and consistency of lactation care, the Lactation Standards Committee of Intermountain Healthcare, a corporation of 23 hospitals, conducted research and analysis over the course of one year to ascertain the best way to improve the quality and consistency of lactation care in their integrated health care system.

Internal time studies were conducted to determine the appropriate allocation of lactation staffing FTEs (full-time equivalents = 40 hours per week).

However, it was determined that it would also be crucial to evaluate, and then standardize, the provision of ALL aspects of lactation care and ensure that all services were provided by the most appropriate staff member and that those staff members had consistent and appropriate training. The evaluation and resulting recommendations were based on:

» Detailed analysis of current staffing allocations, followed by a detailed time study to determine appropriate allocation of FTEs by ancillary personnel, bedside nurses, and the qualified lactation consultant.

» A national survey of 15 hospital-based lactation services across the country to correlate staffing allocations with national recommendations and our time-study findings.

» Assessment of financial impact directly related to lactation failure readmissions resulting in presentations to key insurance payers to improve reimbursement for lactation services and supplies.

» Movement to ensure quality and consistency of staff and patient lactation education.

» Patient satisfaction analysis.

As part of the research, Intermountain Healthcare conducted a survey of 15 hospitals across the United States. A variety of questions were asked regarding their staffing, birth/admission rate, initiation rates, services provided, and key concerns regarding adequacy of lactation-support services. It is interesting to note that, in general, national lactation staffing falls well below published and researched recommendations (see Table 1). These findings agree with the study by Kuan et al. (1999), and they noted the following:

> Although many hospitals have specialized support services for breastfeeding, such as lactation consultants, actual interaction with and support of new mothers may fall consider-ably short of expectations because of staffing patterns and shorter lengths of stay... Signif-icant decreases in nurse staffing as a method of controlling hospital costs may exacerbate these conditions further (Kuan et al., 1999, p. 2, emphasis added).

The Intermountain study provides specific infor-mation and practical steps to hospital(s) that are in the

Table 1. Comparison of National vs. Intermountain Healthcare Lactation Staffing: Allocation of FTEs per Admissions	
Survey Results	**Average FTEs per Admissions**
National survey of Level 2 and 3 hospitals only	1 FTE/1,316.43
Intermountain Health care Level 2 and 3 hospitals only	1 FTE/1,762.87
National survey of all hospitals, including Level 4 facilities	1 FTE/1,060.7
All Intermountain Healthcare hospitals, including Level 4 facilities	1 FTE/1,778.5

process of evaluating their own lactation-support services. If analyzed and structured correctly, lactation services can be shown to reduce overall financial cost to health care organizations, insurance entities, the government, families, and society as a whole. Although the entire study results are not outlined in this article, there are some basic steps that you can take to provide justification for the lactation consultant in your facility.

Step 1: Determine how compliant your state and facility is with the *Healthy People 2020* Breastfeeding Goals using the Breastfeeding Report Card

This report shows how breastfeeding is being protected, promoted and supported in each state using five *outcome* and nine *process* indicators. If possible, quantify your facility's compliance with these same outcome and process indicators.

Step 2: Quantify and report patient satisfaction of hospital lactation care/support

To guide the efforts of inpatient lactation support programs and provide documentation of need for administrators, you need to determine how satisfied or dissatisfied patients are with the current services. A system-wide patient satisfaction survey at the time of discharge is discouraged because of respondent sampling bias and over-surveying patients. Instead, gather data at two- and six-weeks post-discharge from a random sample of discharge patients. Using a professional survey service to conduct and tabulate results is recommended.

Step 3: Analyze Lactation Staffing

Calculate your facility's lactation FTE ratio per births/admissions to determine how close you come to the lactation staffing recommendations in Table 2. Riordan (2005), in discussing the 1:1,000 ratio for hospital-based lactation programs, states:

> This staffing produces a bare minimum coverage that usually results in understaffing and/or part-time coverage. The service—to be effective—should be available seven days a week, on all shifts (p. 41).

To compare against the Intermountain Healthcare staffing recommendations, obtain the following information:

» Annual Newborn Volume: This is the annual newborn birth/admissions (including NICU) to your facility.

» Combined well-baby and NICU breastfeeding initiation rate, and

» Current allocation of FTEs for lactation consultant support.

Table 2. Comparison of Published and Researched Lactation FTE Recommendations

Source	Staffing Ratio Recommendation
Riordan (2005)	3 LCs per 3,000 well born infants
CDC (2009)	1 IBCLC per 1,000 live births
Mannel & Mannel (2006)	**Well born:** 1 FTE/783 breastfeeding couplets **NICU:** 1 FTE/235 infant admits **Well-baby outpatient:** 1 FTE/1,292 breastfeeding couplets discharged **NICU Outpatient:** 1 FTE/818 breastfeeding infants discharged **Education:** 0.1 FTE/1,000 deliveries **Program Development/Administration:** 0.1 FTE/1,000 deliveries **Telephone Follow-up:** 1 FTE/3,915 breastfeeding infants discharged **Research:** 0.1-0.2 FTE total
Intermountain Healthcare Study (2008)[5]	**Mom/Baby Inpatient LC FTE:** Breastfeeding Volume (BFV) x .71/783 = FTE **NICU Inpatient LC FTE:** BFV x .71/235 = FTE **Admin/Program/Education:** .2/1000 births (If a multicenter system, divide FTEs among facilities by % total volumes) **Non-Clinical Support FTE:** Total BFV x .16/1018 **Lactation Follow-Up FTE:** BFV @ discharge/2 then 1:1,292 + 1:818
United States Lactation Consultant Association (2010)	**Level III hospital:** 1.9 FTE lactation consultants per 1,000 births **Level II hospital:** 1.6 FTE lactation consultants per 1,000 births **Level I hospital:** 1.3 FTE lactation consultants per 1,000 births
	NOTE: Each of these recommendations are based on 1 FTE = 40 hours/week.

Step 4: Complete a Basic Calculation

Annual Newborn Volume x Initiation rate/Allocated FTES = FTES/breastfeeding infant.

Further analysis on lactation staffing recommendations has been limited. The only article available that discusses or specifies recommendations for lactation staffing by duty and clinical areas is in an article by Mannel and Mannel (2006). They recommended staffing ratios for all inpatient lactation services, as well as for telephone and outpatient follow-up phone programs. However, Mannel's final calculation formulas do not take into account:

» Level of hospital (acuity/types of patients managed),

» Lactation training level of the bedside nurses, or

» Variations in how lactation consultants use their time and whether or not the tasks performed by these lactation consultants needed to be done by international board certified lactation consultants (IBCLCs).

In order to take those items into account, Intermountain Healthcare conducted two internal time studies at ten hospitals to ascertain work segmentation and what percent of tasks performed by the IBCLC could potentially to be deferred to a non-clinical staff member or a well-trained bedside nurse.

Using this data, FTE calculations were modified to account for service equalization and deferability of task to the appropriate staff member. The Intermountain Healthcare Time Study resulted in recommended adjustments to Mannel and Mannel's FTE calculations based on potential deferability to the correct staff member assuming all other aspects of lactation services were standardized and staff had excellent and consistent training.

The results showed that the Lactation Consultant Service Volume (LCSV) is actually the Breastfeeding Service Volume (BSV) adjusted by the volume of breastfeeding patients that must be managed by an IBCLC. Of tasks done by lactation consultants, 71% *could not* be deferred to the bedside nurse or non-clinician support person.

FTE Calculation Formulas

Mom/Baby FTE: BFV x .71/783 = FTE
NICU FTE: BFV x .71/235 = FTE

Admin/Program/Education: 2/1000 births (If a multicenter system, divide FTEs among facilities by % total volumes)

Non-Clinical Support FTE: Total BFV x .16/ 1018Lactation F/U FTE: BFV @ discharge/2 then 1:1,292 + 1:818 (If a multicenter system, pool F/U FTEs for provision of a regional

---

Terms Defined

Breastfeeding Volume (BFV)

Mom/Baby (M/B) BFV = Births –
NICU admits x % Initiate BF
NICU BFV = Admits x % Initiate BF

Lactation Consultant Service Volume (LCSV)

M/B LCSV = BFV x % non-deferrable tasks
(determined by study)
NICU LCSV = BSV x % non-deferrable tasks
(determined by study)

Follow-Up VOLUME (FUV)

Total discharge # x % BF @ discharge

Step 5: Provide justification to improve financial remuneration for lactation service for those patients with difficult situations requiring an IBCLC

» **Analyze financial tracking options and charge capture**

- Establish a separate tracking code for lactation services so that all expenses and revenue can.

- Standardize your charge/billing forms and billing processes to be in compliance with national billing practices.

- Consider establishing inpatient charges based on the time required for the face-to-face consult, not the acuity, so the charges are the same whether they occurred in the well-baby arena or the NICU.

The assumption is that lactation consultant services are only billed if they are provided by an IBCLC. All other lactation support is provided in the normal standard of care and charges (i.e., room rate).

» **Insurance Buy-In and Reimbursement**

 – With standardized charge/billing forms, billing system, and codes in place, approach key payers in your market. Make appointments with the medical directors of your key insurance providers. The presentation and request should include key information regarding both health and economic benefits of lactation care and support. It is critical that presenters be clinical experts who are well versed in the facts and statistics. If at all possible, it should be a physician-to-physician presentation with a board-certified lactation consultant present and participating in the discussion.

 – It is imperative that requests such as this be made across the country to the large national payers, where it is more difficult to effect change. Local providers are more likely to respond and change their benefit coverage.

Step 6: Determine readmission rates as well as emergency department visits for potential breast-feeding-related complications and the associated financial impact to your hospital and/or organization

Key diagnoses that should be researched are:

» Jaundice

» Dehydration/Hypernatremic dehydration

» Poor weight gain/significant weight loss

» Failure to thrive

Initial readmission rates and costs should be determined prior to implementing lactation-service changes (FTES, education etc.) and again one year after implementation.

Supporting Data

Intermountain Healthcare calculated the financial cost of lactation failure readmissions occurring within 15 days of discharge from one of their 23 hospitals. Data could only be gathered from those infants that were readmitted to their hospitals. Admissions to non-Intermountain hospitals could not be tracked. It was determined that the annual cost to insurers and families for lactation-related readmissions was $ 1.9 million from ONE of our 23 hospitals. A study of 1,385 infants in Madrid from birth to 1 year of age assessed the probability of hospitalization as a result of infectious processes in the first year of life. After estimating the attributable risk, it was found that *30% of hospital admissions would have been avoided for each additional month of full breastfeeding.* Seemingly, 100% of full breast-feeding among 4-month-old infants would avoid 56% of hospital admissions in infants who are younger than 1 year (Paricio Taleyero, 2006, p e92, emphasis added). Meier, Furman, and Degenhardt (2007) noted that the average cost to readmit an infant was $1,163 per day for an average of 3.2 days. Late preterm infants are significantly more likely to require hospital readmission for lactation-related problems. This is in addition to the extra $2,630 incurred for these at-risk babies during the hospital stay.

Conclusion

There are many reasons to improve the quality, consistency, and availability of lactation services.

» **Ethically:** *It is the right thing to do.*

» **Medically:** Research shows that breastfeeding and provision of breast milk are the gold standard, which means that it is critical to have the supports necessary to ensure that mothers and infants are successful at breastfeeding. Also, national organizations state that it is a medical *norm* and expectation to provide consistent and comprehensive lactation services.

» **Financially:** Although lactation services are rarely a money maker, there is potential to charge for the service to offset a portion of those costs. Additionally, provision of effective inpatient lactation care can prevent costly readmissions due to lactation failure(s).

Kuan and colleagues (1999) described the importance of breastfeeding support and access to a lactation consultant as follows:

> In summary, health system support of breastfeeding is an important factor for success, even for highly motivated mothers. This support may include consistent, high-quality information on breastfeeding, and access to a lactation consultant (a credentialed lactation consultant) for all interested mothers. It is important that hospitals develop breastfeeding promotion and support programs and closely monitor outcomes from these services on an ongoing basis (Kuan et al., 1999, p. 10).

References

American Academy of Pediatrics Section on Breastfeeding (2005). Breastfeeding and use of human milk. *Pediatrics, 115*, 496-506.

American Academy of Family Physicians. (2010). *Breastfeeding, family physicians supporting* (position paper). http://www.aafp.org/online/en/home/policy/policies/b/breastfeedingpositionpaper.html

American College of Obstetricians and Gynecologists. (2007). *ACOG calls on ob-gyns, health care professionals, hospitals and employers for increased support for breastfeeding.* http://www.acog.org/About-ACOG/ACOG-Departments/Breastfeeding

Association for Women's Health, Obstetric & Neonatal Nurses. (2010). *Breastfeeding position statement.* http://bit.ly/1M8vqL9

Bartick, M., & Reinhold, A. (2010).The burden of suboptimal breastfeeding in the United States: A pediatric cost analysis. *Pediatrics, 125*, e1048-1056.

Centers for Disease Control and Prevention. (2010). *Breastfeeding.* http://www.cdc.gov/breastfeeding/index.htm

Clegg, S.F., Francis, D.T., & Walker, M. (2008). *Five steps to improving job security for the hospital-based IBCLC.* http://uslca.org/wp-content/uploads/2013/02/5_Steps_To_Improving_Job_Security_for_the_Hospital_Based_IBCLC.pdf

Kuan, L., Britto, M., Decolongon, J., Schoettker, P., Atherton, H., & Kotagal, U. (1999). Health system factors contributing to breastfeeding success. *Pediatrics, 104*(3), e28.

Mannel, R. & Mannel, R. (2006). Staffing for hospital lactation programs: Recommendations from a tertiary care teaching hospital. *Journal of Human Lactation, 22*(4), 409-441.

Meier, P.P., Furman, L.M., & Degenhardt, M. (2007). Increased lactation risk for late preterm infants and mothers: evidence and management strategies to protect breastfeeding. *Journal of Midwifery and Women's Health, 52*(6), 579-587.

Riordan, J. (2005). *Breastfeeding and human lactation, 3rd Ed.;* Sudbury, MA; Jones and Bartlett.

Paricio Talayero, J.M., Lizan-Garcia, M., Otero Puime, A., Benlloch Muncharaz, M.J., Beseler Soto, B., Sanchez- Palomares, M., Santos Serrano, L., & Rivera, L.L. (2006). Full breastfeeding and hospitalization as a result of infections in the first year of life. *Pediatrics, 118*, e92-99.

USLCA (2010). *International Board Certified Lactation Consultant Staffing Recommendations For The Inpatient Setting.* http://www.selca.info/uploads/2/7/0/7/2707925/ibclc_staffing_recommendations_july_20101.pdf

For Further Information

U.S. Breastfeeding Committee (2015). *Healthy people 2020: Breastfeeding objectives.* http://www.usbreastfeeding.org/p/cm/ld/fid=221

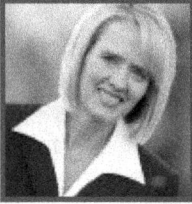

Shannon Francis-Clegg, BSN, MBA, IBCLC, RLC, is a lactation consultant at McKay-Dee Hospital Center. When Shannon began working for Intermountain Healthcare, very few mothers were breastfeeding. Today, about 90 percent of new moms initiate breastfeeding. That's a statistic she is thrilled to report.

Deanne T. Francis, BSN, IBCLC, RLC, MBA, LCCE, is an internal consultant, Lactation Standardization Project of Intermountain Healthcare. She is affiliated with the Utah Valley Regional Medical Center in Provo, Utah.

Breastfeeding Care Satisfaction Survey

Women and Children's Clinical Program

PPQ Questions & Post-Discharge Survey

Intermountain Strategic Planning and Research | October 3, 2007

PPQ Questions

» Did someone in the hospital help you with breastfeeding?

– *If YES*, was that person your nurse or a lactation specialist?

» How well did the (nurse or lactation specialist) explain things to you about breastfeeding?

» How well did the (nurse or lactation specialist) show you how to breastfeed?

6 Weeks Post-Discharge Survey

» Are you still breastfeeding?

– *If YES*, until what age do you intend to breastfeed your baby?

– Are you supplementing with formula?

– *If NO*, are you currently pumping and providing breast milk?

– How old was your baby when you stopped breastfeeding?

– Could you please tell me why you decided to stop breastfeeding?

» Did you receive a breastfeeding booklet called *Living and Learning Together* while in the hospital (This booklet was in your purple discharge folder.)

– *If YES*, how would you rate how helpful this booklet has been?

» Have you had questions or concerns about breastfeeding since you left the hospital?

– *If YES*, did you contact a lactation specialist about your questions or concerns?

» How could we improve the lactation services offered by the hospital?

Recommendations

» Test and refine PPQ questions and post-discharge survey with 10 patients to confirm they are being interpreted as intended.

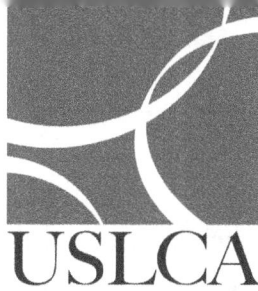

New Taxonomy Codes and the IBCLC

Judy Gutowski, BA, IBCLC, RLC

Keywords: Lactation consultant, non-RN, IBCLC, reimbursement

In 2011, the National Uniform Claim Commission approved a new provider category for non-rn lactation consultants in the U.S. This new code is a Level II Classification under Other Service Providers and Lactation Consultant, Non-RN. *The npi will be useful as the uscla proceeds with efforts to ensure reimbursement for services.*

A new provider category has been established for Non-RN Lactation Consultants, effective April 1, 2011. The National Uniform Claim Commission (NUCC) approved the new code and it was entered into the Taxonomy Code Set in January of 2011. The USLCA Licensure and Reimbursement Committee successfully petitioned the NUCC to include Non-RN Lactation Consultants as a provider category. The RN Lactation Consultant code had already been in existence since 1998.

The RN-Lactation Consultant Code is considered a Level III Area of Specialization, and is listed under the categories of Nursing Service Providers, Registered Nurses, and Lactation Consultants. The numerical index for the code is: 163WL0100X. There is no definition given for the code. The NEW Lactation Consultant, Non-RN, code is listed as a Level II Classification under the category, Other Service Providers and Lactation Consultants, Non-RN. The numerical index for the code is 174N00000X. The definition of the code is:

> An individual trained to provide breastfeeding assistance services to both mothers and infants. Lactation consultants are not required to be nurses and are trained through specific courses of education. The lactation consultant may have additional certification through a national or international organization.
>
> The Taxonomy Code list can be found on
> www.wpc-edi.com/taxonomy.

The taxonomy code set identifies providers based on their separate and distinct roles. Certification and licensure are outside the scope of the code set. The code that has been approved will accommodate lactation consultants who are not registered nurses.

The National Provider Identifier (NPI) is a Health Insurance Portability and Accountability Act (HIPAA) Administrative Simplification Standard. The NPI is a unique identification number for covered health care providers.

Covered health care providers and all health plans and health care clearinghouses must use the NPIS in the administrative and financial transactions adopted under HIPAA. The NPI is a 10-position, intelligence-free numeric identifier (10-digit number). This means that the numbers do not carry other information about health care providers, such as the state in which they live or their medical specialty.

A health care provider is a covered entity if it transmits any health information in electronic form in connection with a transaction for which the Secretary has adopted a standard. For example, any health care provider (individual or organization) who sends electronic health care claims to a health plan(s), is a covered provider and must obtain an NPI. Health care providers who are not covered providers may elect to apply for NPIS, but are not required to do so. Detailed information is available from the Centers for Medicare & Medicaid Services website, http://www.cms.gov/NationalProvIdentStand/

Health care providers can have more than one NPI number and taxonomy associated with their name. For instance, one could have an NPI as an RN Lactation Consultant and a Lactation Consultant, Non-RN.

The taxonomy code set identifies the provider based on their separate and distinct roles. It will be up to the individual to determine the business relationship he or she has when performing lactation consultant duties and which taxonomy code to use. For those IBCLCs who already have the *other service provider* taxonomy code NPI number, you can delete it and replace it with the new NPI for Lactation Consultant, Non-RN. IBCLCs can apply for a new NPI number or update their NPI numbers at this website https://nppes.cms.hhs.gov/NPPES/StaticForward.do?forward=static.npistart

When going through the application process, IBCLCs will choose the categories in the dropdown lists as you see in the diagram. Where the dialogue box asks for you License number, you may put your IBCLC number and state where you reside (not required).

IBCLCs may or may not need an NPI at this time. However, as we proceed with efforts to receive reimbursement for our services as recommended by the *Surgeon General's Call to Action to Support Breastfeeding*, there would be more requirements for the use of the NPI. In addition to having an Individual NPI number, some IBCLCs may have a group number from an organization that employs them.

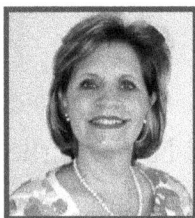

Judy Gutowski, BA, IBCLC, RLC, has worked in the field of lactation since 1989, first as a La Leche League leader and then becoming an International Board Certified Lactation Consultant in 1995. She is currently employed as a lactation consultant in a pediatric practice, where she has the privilege of seeing mothers throughout their breastfeeding experience. She holds a Bachelor of Arts Degree in Psychology. She also spends volunteer time in political and policy advocacy on behalf of mothers and IBCLCs. Her work throughout the U.S., for the United States Lactation Consultant Association, centers on integrating IBCLC services into the healthcare system so that professional, expert breastfeeding support is available to all mothers enabling them to continue breastfeeding as long as they want to do so.

USLCA

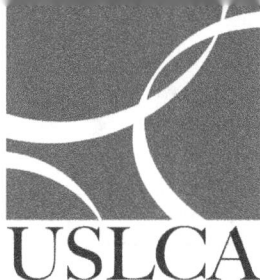

Bfed Texting Program and *Breastfeeding: A Smart Choice* Class
Using Cell Phones to Reach Gen ʏ Mothers

Meg Beard, MPH, MCHES, RD, IBCLC, RLC[1]

Keywords: Breastfeeding, peer counselor, WIC, Gen Y, texting, social media

*Santa Barbara County Public Health Department Nutrition Services and Women, Infants, and Children program in California are meeting the needs of Generation Y mothers through the first of its kind two-way texting program for breastfeeding peer counselor participants called **Bfed**. In addition, there is a prenatal breastfeeding class that has topics that use the phone with apps, video clips that include actual successful breastfeeding peers, and a YouTube channel, to view at a later time. Class participants actually use their cell phones during class instead of having to turn them off.*

---

1   meg.beard@sbcphd.org

For the last 5 years, the breastfeeding coordinator for Women, Infants, and Children (WIC) program has been researching the learning needs of Generation Y (Gen Y) and how to meet them.

Communicating with today's WIC participants has changed. The Millennial or Gen Y is the new face of motherhood. Some basic facts about this cohort include the following:

» Gen Y have birth dates between 1980 and 1994, and go up to around 34 years old.

» They account for 76% of all births, and 85% of first births.

» They trust peers, blogs, and Web communities.

» Texting is their favorite mode of communication.

» Ninety-nine percent of WIC new moms use electronic information resources.

» Ninety-three percent own a cell phone, 79% have unlimited texting, and 55% have a smartphone with Internet service.

» Gen Y mothers want instant gratification and personalization of services, they appreciate diversity, they want to be recognized as multi-dimensional people, and they want to have a voice (Western Region WIC Electronic Technology Project, 2011).

According to Wolynn (2012), "We spend millions of dollars to increase breastfeeding rates. Are we trying too hard or are we just not trying the right way?" Wolynn also states that Gen Y is wired, connected, and jacked in. They are on their computers, tablets, and smartphones sometimes all at the same time. They do not trust traditional media and marketing, and prefer social media. Their most trusted sources and resources are their friends in social media networks. Their most valuable information comes from within this network.

According to the book, *Emerging Theories in Health Promotion Practice and Research*, social-network theory perfectly fits Gen Y members' learning needs (DiClemente, Crosby, & Kegler, 2009, pp. 66–70). Social networks are the go-to channel for information and give the information value and importance. Social networks can be individualized or group-oriented.

Gen Y mothers tend to blend work with their personal life, prefer flexible schedules, relate well to groups, need lots of praise, are used to receiving lots of feedback, expect honesty and fairness, like to have fun, and appreciate explanations (Johnson & Johnson, 2010; Lancaster & Stillman, 2005; Tulgan, 2009).

Our goal was to meet Gen Y mothers where they are using targeted social media via texting. We listened to the needs and desires of our participants, and built our *participant-centered* program from there.

Regarding incorporating cell phones in our health program, we noted the following:

» Use of cell phones and other devices is a current trend in health education.

» Computers are out and the cell phones (mobile devices) are in.

» Mobile devices are the number one consumer product in the world.

Bfed Texting Program

In the spring of 2011, Santa Barbara County's breastfeeding coordinator partnered with Educational Message Services (EMS) located in Ventura, California, to develop, implement, and evaluate a text messaging program for participants in our breastfeeding peer counselor (BPC) program.

EMS is a social marketing and health information technology agency. Prenatal and postpartum text messages were developed by Leanna Moore Watson and translated into Spanish. The Bfed two-way text message program was developed to:

» Meet the communication needs of Gen Y mothers via texting.

» Target social marketing of breastfeeding via texting.

» Increase WIC's local breastfeeding rate.

Automated text messages begin at 12 weeks prenatally, were sent biweekly, and continued weekly starting at Week 26. Occasionally, there were two texts per week. Postpartum mothers also receive two texts per week. Automated texting ends at 10 weeks postpartum. EMS operates the texting platform.

We have developed the *Bfed* name, and short code *893*. Participants have to sign up for the texting program and send back a code word to *opt in*. This means that they agree to receive the texts from WIC's BPC Bfed texting program. EMS runs a private server, having 128-bit encryption that is Health Insurance Portability and Accountability Act–compliant. The program also meets the requirements of the Online Privacy Protection Act, Federal Association of Short Codes, and all cell phone carriers. Texting platforms have stringent requirements and spam texts are against the law.

The Bfed Texting Program is a Web-to-text–based, via cell phone program. The computer Web program sends an automated message at predetermined intervals to the participants' cell phones: one-way communication. This texting program is unique in that it allows for *two-way* interactive communication. (Text4baby is only one way; the recipient cannot text back.)

In our program, participants can actually text back to our two BPCs, Sandra Aguilar Cano and Arely Pulido. The peer counselor can facilitate a dialogue, typing on their office-based computer to the participant who receives the message as a text. Participants like knowing that there is a person at the other end of the text. This helps the texting program feel more personable. Both peer counselors can be on the Web-based program at the same time, responding to their own participants.

Another advantage is that it is easier to type on a keyboard rather than a cell phone. Research indicates that people will say more in a text than on the phone (Evans, Davidson, & Sicafuse, 2013).

Productivity and accuracy are increased. This texting program allows us to collect data on the number of participants, number of texts received, and responses. We think that the Bfed two-way automated breastfeeding texting program is possibly the first in the U.S. and the world. This is a highlight of our BPC program. Are we reaching Gen Y?

Our participants indicated the following:

» *I learned something new in almost all the messages.*

» *There is no need to go to the clinic; all I do is send a text.*

» *I feel very good and more confident about breastfeeding.*

» *When I had my baby, they congratulated me for becoming a mom.*

» *I feel supported because I knew nothing of breastfeeding.*

» *I like receiving the messages. They have great information.*

» *I feel confident and that I am important. Thank you.*

» *I like receiving them. It's a reminder of why breast-feeding is so important and teaches me things I didn't know about.*

» *I enjoy receiving message with information. Because I am a first-time mom, it's nice to know.*

Challenges and lessons learned included the following:

» Peer counselors texting too much and not talking to participants on the phone or in person.

» Data that was lost when peer counselors were texting via cell phone and not texting on the computer.

» Prepaid cell phone cards sometimes do not allow texts.

» Finding funding for the program was difficult.

Box 1. Try the App

Take out your cell phone.

1. Type 898211 where you would put a phone number to text.

2. Text "DEMOEN" for English or "DEMOSP" for Spanish.

3. Press send. (You will receive three actual texts.)

From: Educational Message Services, Inc., Ventura, CA www.educationalmessageservices.com

Call (805) 653-6000 or text "MORE" to 898211.

Other WIC agencies attempting to use this program may encounter additional barriers. These include mothers not being allowed to have cell phones or not being allowed to text, the administration not buying into the importance of texting, and personnel who do not understanding the needs of Gen Y. WIC is on the leading edge in participant-centered counseling. Texting provides personalized attention and increased credibility. The time to start using the capability of cell phones is now because cell phones and texting are here to stay.

Breastfeeding Rates

Breastfeeding rates continue to increase within the BPC program. Data taken from the California Peer Counselor Data Base from October to December 2012 compared to July to September 2013 quarter data showed that peer counselor participants (a subset of WIC participants) had:

» A 28.2% increase in fully breastfeeding rate at 1 month

» A 10% higher fully breastfeeding rate at 3 months

» A 19.6% higher fully breastfeeding rate at 6 months

BPC support, the Bfed texting program, and the early enrollment of infants into the WIC program at age younger than 1 month have helped increase our breastfeeding rates. Most BPC participants in our county are in the Bfed texting program. The peer counselors oversee 8%–10% of all prenatal and postpartum participants on WIC in Santa Barbara County.

Breastfeeding: A Smart Choice, Integrating Smartphone Technology Into a Prenatal Breastfeeding Class

We also decided to revise our prenatal breastfeeding class to reach Gen y mothers, originally inspired to do so after reading an article about Apple founder Steve Jobs. We developed a poster board that looked like a smartphone and referred to the topics as *apps* (Figure 1).

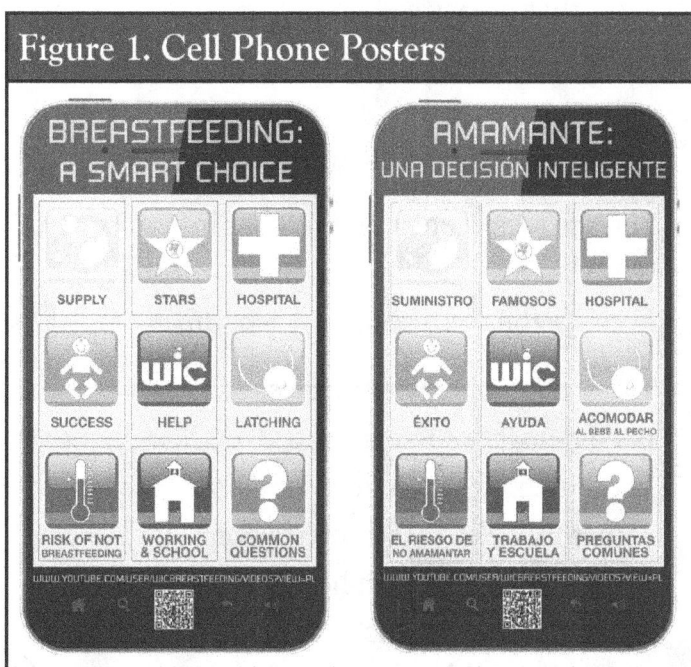

Figure 1. Cell Phone Posters

Source: Keane Ideas Graphic Design and Web Development.

Participants would use their cell phones during class. We used Global Learning Partners' dialogue-based education model and *Learning to Listen, Learning to Teach* trainings, along with an article called *35 Ways to Use an iPhone in a Workshop* (Hodgson, 2010; Vella, 2008). The class is designed to address all types of learning styles: visual, auditory, and kinesthetic. The topics, or apps, were developed from the top questions encountered in Santa Barbara WIC. Gen Y trusts their peers, blogs, or the Web.

Ninety-three percent of mothers own a cell phone, 79% have unlimited texting, and 55% have a smartphone with Internet service. The title of the course itself—*A Smart Choice*—symbolizes that breastfeeding is a smart choice, just like having a smartphone.

This class includes the following:

» The WIC receptionist and teacher instructs participants to take out their cell phones, if they have one, because they will be using them during the class.

» The warm-up activity involves sharing with the person next to them a picture on their phone of their children, an ultrasound photo, a pet, or something else that interests them. If the participant does not have a phone, they are invited to share a picture that is in their wallet or a story about their pregnancy or kids.

» The environment is learner-centered; participants choose what topics, or apps, they want to cover. In a typical class, four to five topics can be covered.

» Because Gen Y mothers tend to trust their peers, two of the apps start with a video of successful

Gen y wic participants who breastfed for a year or who successfully transitioned back to work or school while breastfeeding.

» Our Gen y BPC's cover the *Top 10 Ways to Have a Great Milk Supply*.

» Celebrities who successfully breastfed are highlighted. These people are important to Gen y mothers.

» Some of the apps have participants text themselves if they hear something they want to remember later.

» A popular breastfeeding website is shown. The class also watches a video clip and then practices hand expression.

» For those participants who want to watch the video clips again at a later time, a qr code is provided that takes them directly to the wic YouTube account, where all the clips are available in English and Spanish (Figure 2). The link for this is http://www.youtube.com/user/WICBreastfeeding/videos?view=pl. Participants can access this if they have a smartphone, computer, or at the local library if they do not have a computer.

» The wrap-up includes a review of what they found to be interesting or exciting and how their cell phones can be used to help them breastfeed.

Figure 2. QR Code

We were unable to determine if there was an increase in participants attending these prenatal classes since implementing this program.

Participants are encouraged to attend one prenatal breastfeeding class during the second trimester of pregnancy.

But overall breastfeeding rates for all wic participants at the four main sites have increased using California wic data reporting. (*Fully breastfeeding* is defined for the present article as *formula was not provided at wic*.) The rates are listed in Table 1.

In summary, it is time to provide learner-centered breastfeeding education and reach the needs of Gen y mothers. The cell phone is here to stay, so it should be incorporated into classes and trainings.

Table 1. Breastfeeding Rates for Women, Infants, and Children Participants		
October–December 2011	January–March 2014	% Increase
Fully BF rate at 1 month = 72.36%	84.08%	11.72
Fully BF rate at 3 months = 34.80%	36.29%	1.49
Fully BF rate at 6 months = 24.23%	26.00%	1.77

BF = breastfeeding.

References

DiClemente, R. J, Crosby, R. A., & Kegler, M. C.(2009). *Emerging theories in health promotion practice and research*. San Francisco, CA: Jossey-Bass.

Evans, W. P., Davidson, L., & Sicafuse, L. (2013). Someone to listen: Increasing youth help-seeking behavior through a textbased crisis line for youth. *Journal of Community Psychology*, 41 (4), 471–487.

Hodgson, D. (2010). *35 ways to use an iPhone in a workshop*. Retrieved from: http://www.learningcycle.ca

Johnson, M., & Johnson, L. (2010). Generations, Inc. *From boomers to linksters—Managing the friction between generations at work*. New York, NY: American Management Association Communications.

Lancaster, L. C., & Stillman, D. (2005). *When generations collide: Who they are. Why they clash. How to solve the generational puzzle at work*. New York, NY: Harper Collins.

Tulgan, B. (2009). *Not everyone gets a trophy: How to manage Generation Y*. San Francisco, CA: Jossey-Bass.

Vella, J. (2008). *On teaching and learning: Putting the principles and practices of dialogue education into action*. San Francisco, CA: Jossey-Bass.

Western Region WIC Electronic Technology Project. (2011). Retrieved from http://www.cdph.ca.gov/programs/wicworks/Documents/

Millennial%20Generation/Project%20Information/Western%20
Region%20WIC%20Electronic%20Technology%20Project%20
Abstract.pdf

Wolynn, T. (2012). Using social media to promote and support
breastfeeding. *Breastfeeding Medicine*, 43(5), 364–365.

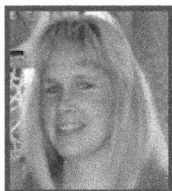

Meg Beard, MPH, MCHES, RD, IBCLC, RLC, has been the
breastfeeding coordinator for Santa Barbara County
Women. Infants, and Children (WIC) program in
California for the last 16 years and chairs and writes
grants for the Santa Barbara County Breastfeeding
Coalition. Santa Barbara County WIC has some of the
highest breastfeeding rates in the state of California.
WIC's caseload is 19,000 with 7 International Board
Certified Lactation Consultants (IBCLC's), 22
lactation educators, and 2 full-time breastfeeding
peer counselors. Santa Barbara County was one
of the first agencies to generate new revenue for
IBCLC visits and the recipient of the California
state WIC *Best Practice Award* in 2003 and 2009. Santa
Barbara County Public Health Department in June
2013 was the recipient of the International Board of
Lactation Consultant Examiners and International
Lactation Consultant Association community
award for excellence and innovation in lactation
care. Breastfeeding is a public health and social
justice issue. Meg Beard resides in Santa Barbara
with her husband and two children who were both
breastfed for 3 years.

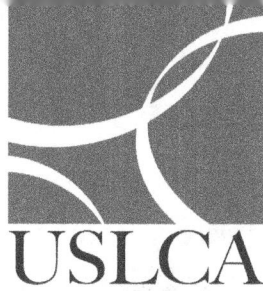

Marketing via the Web and Social Media

Kathleen Lopez[1]

Keywords: Social media, support, breastfeeding, new mothers

Social media is a term that uses Web-based or mobile technologies to facilitate communication and interactive dialogue. Some popular social media sites, such as Facebook, Twitter, or Instagram, have become the go-to sources that mothers use to find breastfeeding support and information. Lactation consultants can use social-media platforms to provide breastfeeding support and information, and reach new mothers in their communities. These platforms can also be useful when mothers want to have the support of other new mothers, but are limited by geography or timezone.

---

1   Kathleen Lopez is a student lactation consultant and aspiring IBCLC

More than ever before, the world is truly at our fingertips. *Let your fingers do the walking* no longer refers to that giant book that immediately makes its way to the recycling bin, but to the world of always-on information that is available to us with a click of the mouse and the touch of a pad. As lactation consultants, we have the unique opportunity to use online and social-media channels to both reach and support our clients. While there are many breastfeeding issues that require an in-person consultation, there are also many that do not. The use of the Web and social media in an IBCLC's practice should serve to consolidate the accurate, reliable, and current information on breast-feeding. Used wisely, social media can act as a valuable back-up assistant.

What is *Social Media*?

The term *social media* refers to the use of Web-based and mobile technologies to turn communication into an interactive dialogue.

For IBCLCs, it's a way to use these technologies and channels to engage directly with clients, as well as other lactation professionals and maternity-care providers. It is dynamic, existing in real time, and is constantly updated, just like an ongoing conversation. It's also extremely popular; a 2009 Pew study examining how people access the Web specifically for health-related information showed that up to 42% of adults searching for this information online say that they, or someone they know, have been helped once they've followed medical advice found on the Internet. This number is almost double the same statistic from just three years earlier, and as of this writing, Facebook alone has over 800 million active users.

What does this have to do with my practice as an IBCLC?

According to Scott Public Research, Generation x and Generation y women tend to rely on the Web and peer contact for their information needs. Scott also shows that the younger adult generation simply does not pay attention to more traditional forms of health marketing promotion.

Women who use social media on a daily basis often turn to it as their first line of defense. Perhaps more importantly, these generations are often doubtful of advice that comes to them from outside their realm of social contact. Younger, socially savvy mothers may be more willing to listen to their peers than seek the advice of an older, more experienced lactation professional.

So where do I start?

Let's take a quick quiz. Where do you look first when seeking information or professional services? Draw a mental circle around all that apply, and then think about where your clients or other local new mothers might be looking for information and support. It may be very different than what you think!

Is the list longer than you thought? Did some of the items surprise you? It is interesting to note that *more than*

421 *hospitals* have YouTube channels, and that companies that make products for the mothers you serve are on Twitter, Facebook, or have blogs. Consider the amount of time it takes for a mother to get the information or support she needs. Without quick turnaround, a mother may feel unsupported. Those lonely, isolated overnight hours can leave a new mother feeling especially vulnerable. More and more, they are using iPads or laptops to find information and support that they need.

Word of mouth	Phone book	Internet search	Reference book/ magazine	Journal publications
Facebook	Twitter	Blog posts	Chat rooms or instant messaging	Message boards
Telephone hotline	YouTube videos	SMS text messaging	iPhone/iPad or Android app	Webinar

If your clients can reach a part of you after hours, chances are they will feel a deeper connection to you and your practice, and as a result, will feel more supported. Don't forget, that to a new mother with breastfeeding issues, every question can feel like an emergency. Waiting even three or four hours for an answer can be an eternity. Through the use of online channels, such as Facebook and

Twitter, or dedicated informational Web pages and apps, IBCLCs can provide searchable answers or have quick, direct engagement that takes less time than a phone call or office visit. Perhaps most importantly, we can disseminate information, gain visibility for the IBCLC credential, and add commentary to (and sometimes even correct) information that already exists.

While the ever-changing landscape of technology can at times seem overwhelming, it is important to remember that reaching new mothers is most effective when we engage them in the places where they are asking questions.

For Further Information

http://en.wikipedia.org/wiki/social_media

http://www.facebook.com/press/info.php?statistics

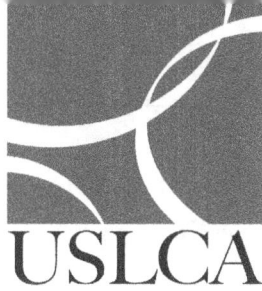

Connecting With Today's Mothers:
Breastfeeding Support Online

Lara Audelo, CLEC[1]

Keywords: Breastfeeding, social media, blogging, Facebook, Generation x, Millennials

Since the mid-1990s women have been using the Internet to offer breastfeeding support to one another. As technology has rapidly changed, mothers have kept up with the pace and found ways to embrace the changes, using them to their advantage. It is essential for all who work with breastfeeding mothers in a professional capacity to understand the generational differences that exist, oftentimes between mothers and providers. For lactation professionals, it is valuable to know how mothers use the Internet, and the platforms they are using for breastfeeding support. Whether it is through social media platforms or blogging, lactation professionals

1   mamapeardesigns@gmail.com

have more ways than ever before to help mothers by offering their expertise in online settings.

In the last two decades we have watched the Internet transform our culture in countless ways. Cyberspace has proven to be an extremely powerful tool that we have been able to harness, allowing people to connect in new ways, and therefore, collaborate in great numbers and across great distances. Perhaps one of the best examples is in the support that women give one another with respect to pregnancy, breastfeeding, and parenting. Today's uniquely interactive social media platforms and devices, such as smartphones, give mothers greater access to valuable online breastfeeding help. Because women are turning online in record numbers, it is important that lactation professionals meet these mothers where they are, whether it is through blogs, Facebook, Twitter, or other popular social media sites.

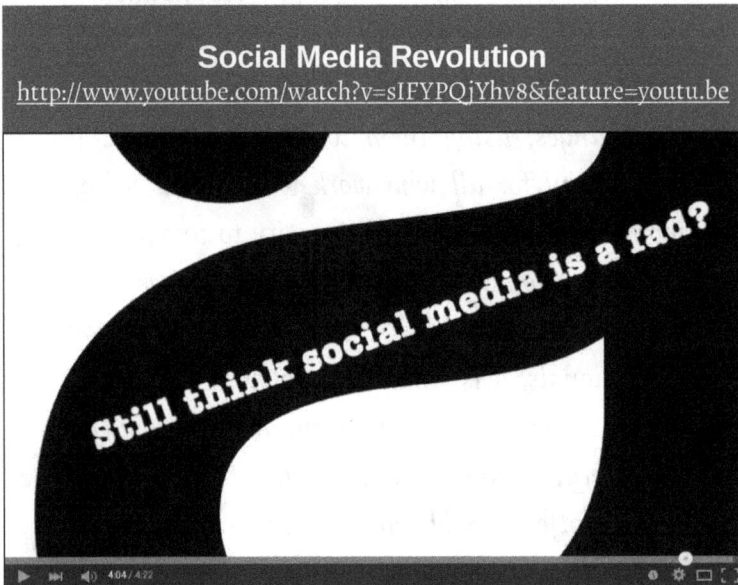

Social Media Revolution
http://www.youtube.com/watch?v=sIFYPQjYhv8&feature=youtu.be

Still think social media is a fad?

A Brief History of Online Breastfeeding Support

With respect to breastfeeding support, the first women to use the Internet for this purpose did so through listservs and email loops in the mid-1990s.

Small groups of women reached out, often lacking assistance in their own local communities and social circles, to others who were in the same place in life as they were: breastfeeding their babies and navigating the uncharted waters of motherhood.

One of the first listservs formed, by an international cohort of breastfeeding mothers, was called Parent-L. Today, as the creators and original members of Parent-L have gone from being mothers to grandmothers, and from using a listserv to a private Facebook group to maintain their relationships, they realized that they paved the way for women connecting via digital technology.

Almost two decades ago, establishing a website, or even starting a listserv, was not something that just anyone could do. Hanna Graeffe, a Parent-L member from Finland, recently recognized by one of the largest baby magazines in her country as an online pioneer of breastfeeding support, noted it was necessary to know someone from a university to establish a listserv (Audelo, 2013).

When we look at the legacy of listservs (Parent-L, BFAR, LACTNET), they offered more than just breastfeeding support. Many of these women emerged as leaders in the field of lactation. They wrote the books and articles that we use, and they became key players in breastfeeding initiatives around the world. Graeffe shared that in Finland:

> The National Breastfeeding Association started forming and growing from that list, and now the association has several employees, and a position as the breastfeeding expert in this country; There are plenty of support groups, both real-life and online available, as well as a national phone line you can call for breastfeeding support. All this came from the breastfeeding email list (Audelo, 2013, p.21)!

Mothers in need took this new technology, which did not offer today's intuitive and user-friendly interfaces, and mastered it, for their own benefit, and to help other mothers.

As is true in today's online communities, there was a regular flow of information back and forth. Anthropologist, Kathy Dettwyler, was an original Parent-L member. She stated,

> Remember, by the time the Internet came along, I had nursed three kids and spent my career doing research on breastfeeding, including speaking at conferences, and writing articles and books. I was the one providing support. I set up a website, with lots of articles and links (Audelo, 2013, p.20).

Mothers who connect online with each other today, whether through blogs, Facebook, or Twitter, can trace the foundation of these networks back to the listservs and women who were the online pioneers in breast-feeding support.

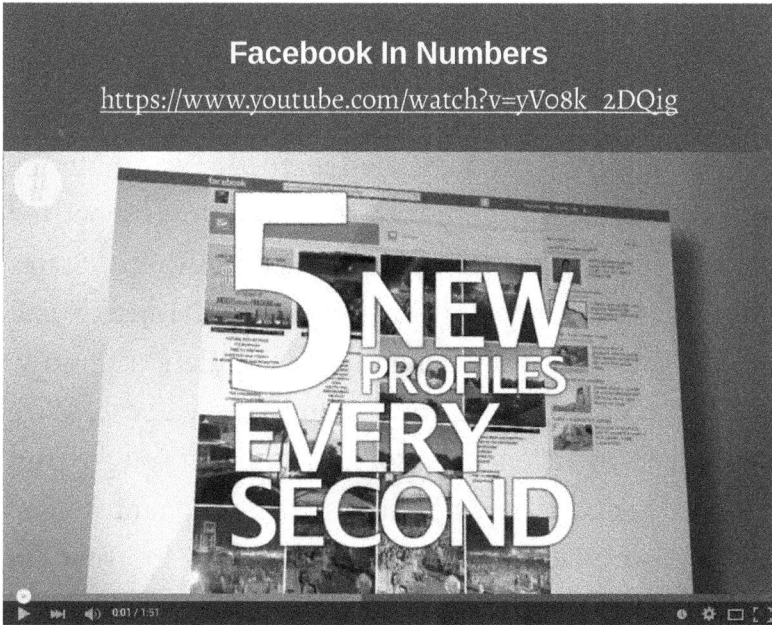

Facebook In Numbers
https://www.youtube.com/watch?v=yVo8k_2DQig

Understanding Generational Differences

Our ages often have a direct effect on the rate at which we embrace new technology, and on our ability to adopt change. Baby boomers have witnessed the swift techno-logical changes that have occurred in the past few decades, and often feel overwhelmed by what they need to learn.

In contrast, Generation x and Millennials have grown up with technology, and became connected at an early age. The online queries of the Generation xers and Millennials do not just go online to look up recipes for dinner or map out directions; they seek answers to some of their most personal questions online.

Kathryn Zickuhr (2010) studied these three generations and their use of the Internet, and found that searching for health information, an activity that was once the primary domain of older adults, is now the third most popular online activity for all Internet users 18 and older. A study published in 2009, examining the sociodemographic and health-related factors associated with current adult social media users in the United States, found that the potential for impacting the health and health behavior of the general U.S. population through social media is tremendous (Chou et al., 2009). With medical information being some of the most sought-after knowledge online, it is no surprise that pregnant women and new mothers might also find digital information about all things related to motherhood to be valuable.

It is important that we know how each generation uses the Internet, because that knowledge helps us figure out the nuances of how the younger mothers prefer to be addressed, and how they like to obtain information. Diana West, IBCLC, author, and co-founder of BFAR.org, was among the first wave of mothers to use the Internet for support in the 1990s. She recognizes the differences among the generations. West highlights that today's mothers are increasingly Millennials, but most practices are in danger of becoming outdated because they are geared toward Generation-x mothers. When lactation professionals understand what motivates the Millennials, they will be best able to help them. What we are seeing in many cases, and partly because Millennial mothers are quick and eager to share their opinions, is that the younger, socially savvy mothers may be more willing to listen to their peers than seek the advice of an (older, more experienced) lactation professional (Lopez, 2012, p.39). If this is the case, how can we make sure that the lactation professional remains a vital part of the support network?

Embracing the Change

Social media is an ever-changing phenomenon, and many feel that they are just scratching the surface.

> We are at the age where we need to be wired for new technologies, as well as being able to speak the shorthand defining each new medium (Breheny, 2011, p.3).

Online support communities have been around for more than 20 years, and are clearly not a fad. Lactation professionals need to understand online support if they are want to reach mothers where they are today.

> While the ever-changing landscape of technology can at times seem overwhelming, it is important to remember that reaching new mothers is most effective when we engage them in the places where they are asking questions (Lopez, 2012, p. 40).

Recognizing the changing times, the United States Breastfeeding Committee (USBC) called on IBCLCs to embrace social media and use it as a way to disseminate accurate, evidence-based information (McCann & McCulloch, 2012).

In her *Call-to-Action* in 2011, Dr. Regina Benjamin, the former u.s. Surgeon General, noted that social media was an important tool for reaching breastfeeding mothers (McCann & McCulloch, 2012).

To truly understand the reach of social media, we must recognize that Facebook, the most popular and widely used platform, has over one billion users, and three-quarters of those access the site through their mobile devices (Constine, 2013). The Internet is not just a place to visit for information. It is participative, highly interactive, and for over a billion people worldwide, an integral part of daily life. We should not discount the value of face-to-face interaction, of course, but for many women, the introduction to breastfeeding and the lactation professional comes by way of social media: a blog, Facebook page, or Twitter account.

As such, the opportunity exists for mothers to reach reliable information from professionals on these platforms. Hopefully, we see how important social media is to women of childbearing age, and are aware of the value in supporting women through these channels.

Blogs

All social media platforms vary in their appeal, but blogs are to be noted as an especially valuable resource for professionals and mothers. Blogging allows professionals to share their information with a wider audience than they can reach locally. Mothers can access the information when it is convenient for them. The statistics prove that blogs are sought-after resources, with 81% of mothers reporting that blogs help build confidence about parenting skills, and 67% use them as a primary source of parenting advice (McCann & McCulloch, 2012). Robin Kaplan, an IBCLC in private practice, found that her blog filled this exact need.

> While there is never a shortage of content when it comes to breastfeeding, there are plenty of bad articles about breastfeeding on the Internet. My goal is to write articles that offer evidence-based recommendations in a non-judgmental way, for mothers to refer to in years to come (Audelo, 2013, p.176).

It is critical to provide evidence-based information for those mothers who are searching. Some women never seek breastfeeding advice in person—for a variety of reasons, ranging from monetary constraints to geographical limitations—but they might just meet their breastfeeding goals with information online. There are likely countless women who owe their breastfeeding success to their online support communities.

Formula Companies are Also Adept at Social Media

Additionally, it is worth noting that companies, ranging from the largest infant formula companies to small businesses selling unique, even homemade, baby products and wares, use social media constantly to reach mothers. These companies know where moms are, and have chosen to meet them online. The infant formula industry is quite adept at orchestrating and executing savvy social media campaigns, which all offer a wide array of infant-feeding advice, including breastfeeding information. These companies, with huge advertising budgets, spend millions annually, knowing that if they offer breastfeeding advice, they can reach mothers.

They often promote their help hotlines through social media, or sponsor prominent advertisements on popular blogs with large followings of mothers. The top hits on a Google search for breastfeeding, which yields over 26 million results in less than half a second, are from the websites of formula companies. How many mothers have clicked on one of those links that offers breastfeeding advice, only to be bombarded with advertisements that promote formula?

And it doesn't stop there. Formula companies offer free smartphone applications, and sponsor Twitter parties that offer prize products. McCulloch and McCann (2013) suggest that lactation professionals acting as advocates for breastfeeding mothers must not only keep up with technological changes, but also seize the opportunities that social media offers in terms of engaging in meaningful conversations that will affect positive change.

Today's Mothers: Digital Natives

Generation-x and Millennial mothers are digital natives, so it stands to reason that they spend more time online once their babies are born. Statistics show that time spent using the Internet increases by as much as 44 percent after giving birth; additionally, 71% of parents are Facebook users, and 81 percent are mothers (McCulloch & McCann, 2013). If mothers are going online for health information, is it because they are not able to obtain answers to their questions from their health care providers?

Perhaps providers are not wholly aware of their patients' desire for more health information (Gray, 2013, p.7). Some of the most frequently asked questions in online settings *are about initial feeding decisions and the need for providers to address stress-related feeding problems* (Gray, 2013, p.7).

If this is the case, then we can assume the mothers need lactation professionals to fill this void for them. If they are not talking to health care providers, then where are they finding valuable, reliable, evidence-based information about these critical issues and questions?

> Through the use of online channels, such as Facebook and Twitter, or dedicated informational Web pages and apps, IBCLCs can provide searchable answers or have quick, direct engagement that takes less time than a phone call or office visit ... Used wisely, social media can act as a valuable back-up assistant (Lopez, 2012, p.40).

It is not only beneficial for lactation professionals to use social media for the purpose of supporting mothers and babies, but doing so also has great potential benefits for business, whether it is private practice, hospital, or clinic.

A wonderful example of professionals and mothers working together to foster mother-to-mother support, and valuable resources in local communities, is through breast-feeding awareness events. The Big Latch On, which has been held the last few years during World Breastfeeding Week in August, is a gathering that serves mothers and professionals alike. Aimed at increasing awareness, the event owes its grassroots marketing success to social media.

Mothers have embraced and promoted it through various platforms, and as a result, turnout sets record numbers. Events such as these help lactation professionals connect with local individual women and groups, all the while using the global social media network to promote and protect breastfeeding.

We do not know exactly how many lactation profes-sionals there are who use social media regularly, as there has yet to be any data published. According to the Interna-tional Lactation Consultant Association (ILCA), there are over 13,200 IBCLCs in the United States. ILCA's Facebook page has over 8,500 followers, but that number includes all Facebook users (mothers, volunteer breastfeeding supporters, and professionals), not just IBCLCs.

It is probably safe to say there are many IBCLCs who do not have a social-media presence. This number will increase as more Baby Boomers adopt social media, and as Gen xers and Millenials assume the torch passed to them from the older generation of lactation professionals. These mothers will encourage all lactation professional to embrace *significant changes in the way we promote and [support] breastfeeding ... [including] the adoption of new and emerging technologies* (Heinig, 2009, p. 263).

Conclusion

Social media is, in effect, a new language that we have to learn to speak, as without it we risk the inability to make initial connections with future generations of breastfeeding mothers.

We must remember who our target audience is, where they are, what they are looking for, and how they prefer to be engaged. Just as important, we cannot neglect the fact that to promote breastfeeding and the profession, IBCLCs need to be willing to use social media to stay informed and up-to-date with current events relevant to the profession, stay connected to their colleagues, and to help inform mothers with reliable information. Lactation professionals do not have to master every platform, or have a presence on every social media site.

But working to bridge the technology gap, at your own comfort level, is vital to keeping touch with today's moms. The Internet serves to introduce lactation professionals to mothers who need your expertise, and a social media presence provides a way for you to connect.

It is evident that in 2013, mothers have built their villages online as support networks that are often closely knit, and are rarely static. We need to know where they are, meet them there, and be willing to offer the support they need, in ways they grasp.

References

Audelo, L. (2013). *The virtual breastfeeding culture: Seeking mother to mother support in the digital age.* Amarillo, TX: Praeclarus Press.

Breheny, D. (2011). *Using web technologies in lactation healthcare promotion.* Retrieved from http://www.slideshare.net/brehenyd/using-web-technologies-for-the-lactation-professional

Chou W.S., Hunt Y.M., Beckjord E.B., Moser R.P., & Hesse B.W. (2009). Social media use in the United States: Implications for health communication. *Journal of Medical Internet Research, 11*(4), e48, doi: 10.2196/jmir.1249

Constine, J. (2013). *Facebook's growth since IPO in 12 big numbers.* Retrieved from http://techcrunch.com/2013/05/17/facebook-growth/

Gray, J. (2013). Feeding on the web: Online social support in the breastfeeding context. *Communications Research Reports, 30*(1), 1-11.

Heinig, J. (2009). Breastfeeding promotion for generations X and Y: Why the old ways won't work. *Journal of Human Lactation. 25*(3), doi: 10.1177/0890334409341450

Lopez, K. (2012). Marketing via the web and social media. *Clinical Lactation.* 3(1), 39-40. Retrieved from http://www.ingenta-connect.com/content/springer/clac/2012/00000003/00000001/art00009;jsessionid=245dpss83c2rc.alexandra

McCann, A. D., & McCulloch, J. E. (2012). Establishing an online and social media presence for your IBCLC practice. *Journal of Human Lactation, 28*(4), doi: 10.1177/0890334412461304

McCulloch, J.E. & McCann, A.D. (2013). *Defeating the formula death star, one tweet at a time: Using social media to advocate for the WHO code.* Retrieved from http://www.scienceandsensibility.org/?s=-jeanette+mcculloch

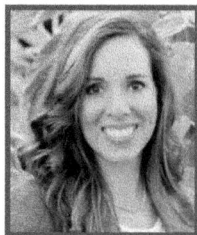

Lara Audelo, CLEC, is the mom of two young boys, and is passionate about raising awareness for breastfeeding and supporting mothers and babies in meeting their breastfeeding goals. She believes increased education for all is key to supporting moms and that online breastfeeding support is fast becoming a critical tool for helping mothers achieve their infant feeding goals. A breast-feeding mom for more than seven years, she received her Certified Lactation Education Counselor (CLEC) credential from University of California, San Diego.

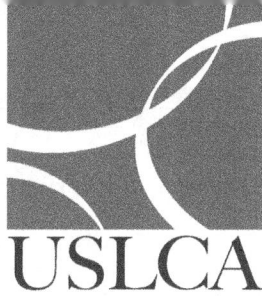

Taking My Private Practice Paperless

Jessica Lang Kosa, PhD, IBCLC, RLC[1]

Keywords: Electronic records, paperless, IBCLC, lactation support

IBCLCs in private practice may find that going paperless may help them with charting, records, communications, and care plans. Paperless record keeping may also help integrate client emails with other client records, and may ease billing and client follow-up. This article describes some of the tools that are helpful in making the transition to paperless and what must be done to ensure the security and confidentiality of client records.

I'm writing this in the YMCA lobby while my daughter is in swim class. As an independent International Board Certified Lactation Consultant (IBCLC) working in a solo

1   jesskosa@gmail.com

private practice and the mother of three, I need to use these little chunks of time. This was one of my main goals when I decided to change my practice to a *paperless* one. Being paperless means that all of my charting, records, communications, and care plans are recorded on one of my electronic devices. I have an hour while she swims. I have emails from clients with questions. I want to check their records before responding to them, even if it's just to make sure I know the baby's name and age. Having a paperless practice gives me access to my records via my phone or iPad.

One of the strongest reasons for making this switch was the need to combine emails with the rest of my client records. Nearly all of my clients do email me at some point, and I wanted to integrate a record of those communications in the client's chart. Printing out emails and stapling them to the consult report seemed tedious and wasteful. Making the whole record electronic solved that problem.

Other IBCLCs may consider going paperless for many reasons: avoiding paper waste, saving storage space, and making communication with clients and other providers easier are also benefits. I've also seen many different ways of approaching a paperless practice.

Here is what I did; I have my clients fill out an online intake form and sign my consent form. For this, I use FormSite. I already had an account because I use it for registration for my breastfeeding classes. It's web-based so it can be used by anyone regardless of what type of computer they have. An alternative would be to have an intake form built into your website. But for many, any changes would require having to pay to have updates made by the person who runs your website. FormSite has a secure server feature, allowing for Health Insurance Portability and Accountability Act (HIPAA)-compliant collection of protected information. These features required a paid account on FormSite, but you can get a basic account for free to try it out.

Building my intake form using their interface was time consuming, but not difficult. It allows you to drag and drop questions of different types (checkbox, multiple choice, text answer, date), as well as arrange and format them. I built in my consent form and HIPAA notice as well. When a client makes an appointment, I give her the link and password to access the form. If she didn't have Internet, I'd go back to a paper form, but it's only happened once. When she fills it out, the site sends me an e-mail notification. I log into FormSite and download the info as a spreadsheet.

Then the fun begins!

Once I receive their intake form, I paste the spreadsheet, including the intake information, into an application called Bento—this is a Mac-based program. If you have a PC, you would paste it into Excel or whatever spreadsheet program you like. I chose Bento because it was the only application I found that would combine e-mails, spreadsheet data, photos, and files all together.

Now, when a client e-mails to say that the baby is up to 8 lb, I can drag the email into her record in Bento.

If she sends me a picture, ditto. Also, her care plan and pediatrician's report will be in there too. At the actual consult, I use Bento on an iPad. It syncs with my home computer. Important note: it syncs over my own home network—not through the Cloud. The question of HIPAA compliance and the Cloud remains formally unanswered, so I feel it behooves me to keep clinical info out of the Cloud. (Yes, unencrypted email is also a potential HIPAA concern, so I address that in my consent form. And I don't text with clients at all, except about scheduling.) Bento allows me to create forms on my iPad to visually organize info. I have one form that shows the intake info she gave me online, one with her doctors' contact info, one for the evaluation I do at the consult, one for follow-up info, and one for my superbill.

I use checkboxes and dropdown menus as much as possible so that I spend minimal time typing. I complete the evaluation form as I go along during the consult. At the end, I complete the superbill, which I will export as a PDF file to send her. The follow-up form will contain her care plan and report (as PDF files), emails, notes on phone calls, or any subsequent visits. The providers' form is linked to a database of doctors so I can easily look up their phone or fax numbers.

Another nice aspect of this is—by using checkboxes—I can easily quantify data across my whole practice, such as what percentage of babies I referred for tongue-tie. I could create Bento forms for my reports and care plans, but I haven't. Bento doesn't allow for a lot of formatting.

I like them to be in letter form, so I do those separately using Pages (Mac's word processor). I save the care plan and report a PDF file. I email the care plan to the client, along with her superbill and any handouts or additional info I want to send her. I use PamFax (there are many other choices for online faxing) to fax the report to the pediatrician and OB/GYN.

With all-electronic records, backup is critical. I use Carbonite for remote backup (if my house burns down or if my computer is stolen) and Time Machine for easy local backup (if my computer freaks out). Both backups happen automatically. All of this takes some investment of time to get up and running, but I've definitely found that it makes my practice run more smoothly.

Reprinted from the Lactation Matters blog, May 21, 2013. Used with permission. **Author's Note:** The Bento app referred to in this post is scheduled to be discontinued and may no longer be available at publication time. To learn about and discuss various paperless systems IBCLCs are using, join the Yahoo group Paperless IBCLC at http://groups.yahoo.com/neo/groups/paperlessIBCLC/info

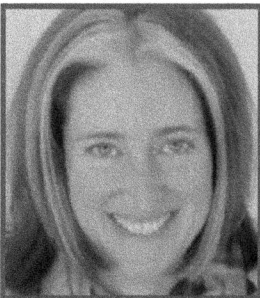

Jessica Lang Kosa is an International Board Certified Lactation Consultant in private practice in the Boston area. She offers home visits for comprehensive breastfeeding help and teaches courses in breastfeeding support for professionals who work with mothers and babies.

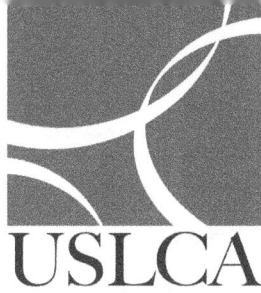

Caring for Ourselves When Caring for Others

What Lactation Consultants Need to Know about Burnout and Compassion Fatigue

Kathleen Kendall-Tackett, PhD, IBCLC, RLC, FAPA[1]

Keyword: Compassion fatigue, burnout, lactation consultants, caregiver stress

Caregiving is rewarding, but can come at high cost to the care provider. Our field started with a dedicated group of volunteers who wanted to make a difference for mothers and babies, and who were willing to do whatever it took to meet these needs. Unfortunately, that same willingness often made us vulnerable to both burnout and compassion fatigue. Giving our time and skills to others is a noble goal. But caring for others must always be balanced with self-care. If we do not practice self-care, we are in

1   kkendallt@gmail.com

danger of becoming impaired. To be our best, and to give the best to the families we serve, we must be willing take care of ourselves too.

A couple of weeks ago, I had a major *Ah-ha* moment. I first spoke with a colleague who is a great grass-roots champion of breastfeeding. She had recently attended a meeting of her local breastfeeding coalition, and was shocked to see how beaten-down and discouraged the members were. Shortly after this conversation, I attended a webinar on burnout and compassion fatigue that affects people in caregiving roles. In this webinar, trauma experts, Charles and Kathleen Figley described why caregivers need to take time to care for themselves.

Burnout can be described as a state of physical, emotional, and spiritual exhaustion brought on by too many demands, not enough support and recognition, job insecurity, and work that seems so overwhelming that you can never feel like you are doing a good or thorough job. Its onset is frequently gradual and insidious. In contrast, compassion fatigue can happen quickly. It occurs when caregivers witness something in the course of their duties that is highly traumatic, such as seeing another care provider traumatize a mother through their actions.

Burnout and compassion fatigue are not issues we have addressed for lactation consultants, but need to. Think about it; Many of you are fighting uphill battles at your institutions. You are frequently the only ones doing the work, so that you may feel overwhelmed by your responsibilities. Many of you are in danger of losing your jobs because the skills you offer are not valued. You get labeled as a fanatic (or worse) because you care about mothers and babies. And then there is the issue of pay... In addition, you may have witnessed mothers and babies being harmed by another provider at your institution. In some ways, the history of our field may be partially to blame.

Many of us initially came into lactation as volunteers. We worked with mothers and babies because we loved it and wanted to make a difference. I started my work in lactation as a volunteer. I was a La Leche League leader for 18 years, and took on many roles in my capacity as a Leader, eventually becoming the Area Coordinator of Leaders for LLL of Maine and New Hampshire, and serving on the international board of directors.

I've spoken at LLL conferences throughout the U.S. and Canada, and in many other parts of the world. I have seen first-hand the amazing work these volunteers have done. The world would be far worse had it not been for these volunteers. In addition, without those volunteers, we would not have lactation consultants.

Unfortunately, our willingness to step in has come at a high cost: devaluing ourselves and not practicing regular self-care. Because we cared so much, we often did whatever it took to meet the needs of mothers and babies, and that often meant being willing to work without pay, or even basic resources. For example, I know many La Leche League Leaders who had bakesales or car washes to buy copies of *Medications and Mothers' Milk* for all their local doctors (great activity, but what's wrong with that picture? Why can't the doctors buy their own books). A lot of people in our field are working to change the compensation that lactation consultants receive. But until they do, *we* need to value the time we spend in helping mothers, whether we are paid or volunteer.

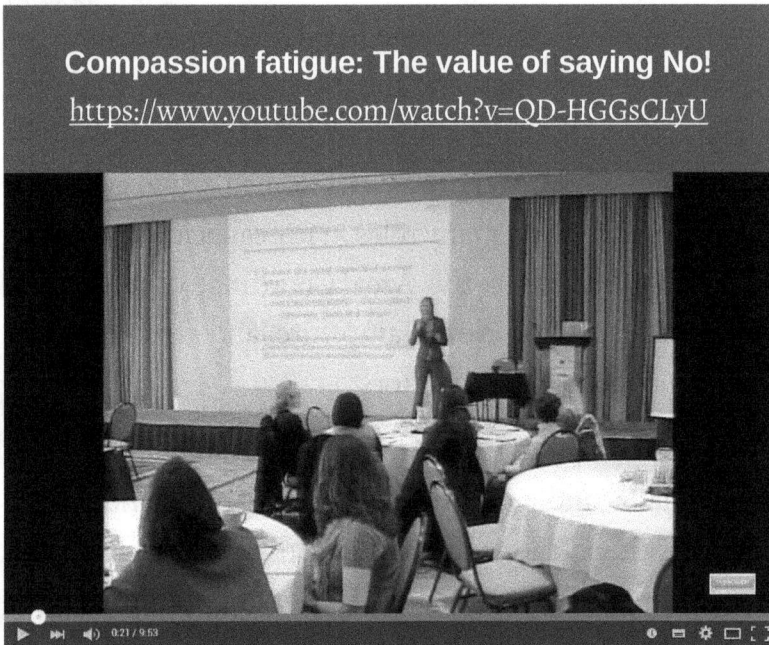

Compassion fatigue: The value of saying No!
https://www.youtube.com/watch?v=QD-HGGsCLyU

People with burnout or compassion fatigue, often try to compensate for the emotional difficulties they are facing by throwing themselves into their work. They try to multitask their unhappiness away by doing several things at once (e.g., eating lunch while catching up on case files). Unfortunately, the work is never done. They may also cut out activities that might rejuvenate them, such as exercise, or spending time with family and friends.

The result of burnout or compassion fatigue is often depression, anger, blaming, a diminished sense of personal accomplishment, exhaustion, hopelessness, irritability, sleep disturbances, and cynicism, which can lead to substance abuse or other self-destructive activities. If any of this sounds familiar, you are not alone. Burnout or compassion fatigue are NOT character flaws. People who care the most are often the ones most prone to them.

It is here that we must heed the lessons learned in the trauma field: trauma workers cannot sustain their work if they are not diligent about their own needs. In fact, a caregiver who does not practice self-care can become *impaired*. So we owe it to ourselves, and the women we serve, to become aware of these issues, listen to what trauma workers have to say, and make self-care a priority.

Lessons from the Trauma Field

According to trauma expert, Charles Figley, we need to make a specific commitment to self-care. He said that we should **first do no harm to ourselves when helping others.** Second, we need to attend to our physical, social, emotional, and spiritual needs as a way of ensuring high-quality services to those who look to us for support.

Figley recommends that we make a formal, tangible commitment to our self-care. Put it in writing. Set deadlines and goals for self-care activities. Develop specific strategies for letting go of work in off-hours. We need to embrace rejuvenation activities that are fun, stimulating, inspiring, and that generate joy. We also need to set tangible goals for getting adequate rest, exercising, and eating well. We need to set reasonable limits on what we take on. Practice saying *no* once in a while, and don't be so quick to volunteer for everything. Let someone else have a turn. (I know it's hard, but you can do it!)

Find supportive people, particularly peers. Find a self-care buddy and hold each other accountable. If your local or state breastfeeding coalitions are suffering from burnout or compassion fatigue, maybe you can address these issues as a group. You can also join with local and national groups, such as USLCA, to advocate for the pay you deserve. Finally, know when to ask for help. Charles Figley, in talking about disaster relief following Hurricane Katrina, noted the following.

> The main thing with regard to self-care is that those who are selfless and compassionate have an Achilles heel—they don't pay enough attention to themselves. So we have to save them from themselves ... The people who are drawn to [social work] are extraordinarily vulnerable to compassion fatigue. The same is true for the faith community, for nurses, even certain specialties within the military, and Red Cross volunteers. There's a tendency to be selfless and to help other people. So they have to recognize that they're more vulnerable than most people because they neglect their own needs. http://www.medscape.com/viewarticle/513615

In short, self-care is not selfish. It's the thing that will allow you to continue in this work.

Let's all resolve to practice self-care in the year to come. And let's hold each other accountable to make positive changes in our lives. Valuing ourselves and our time will be good for us and improve the care we provide. It's the ultimate win-win.

See also the Caregiver's Bill of Rights
http://www.healthycaregiving.com/pages/TheBillOfRights.pdf

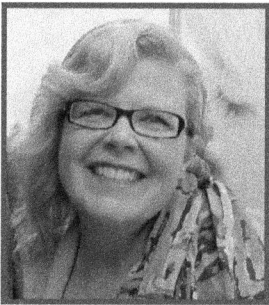

Kathleen Kendall-Tackett, PhD, IBCLC, RLC, FAPA, is a health psychologist, IBCLC, and Fellow of the American Psychological Association. Dr. Kendall-Tackett is Editor-in-Chief of *Clinical Lactation,* clinical associate professor of pediatrics at Texas Tech University Health Sciences Center, and owner of Praeclarus Press www.PraeclarusPress.com.

USLCA

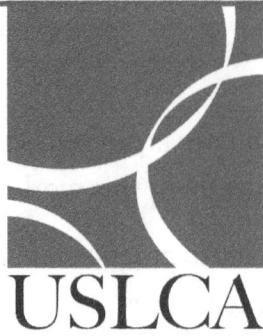

USLCA is a non-profit membership association focused on advancing the International Board Certified Lactation Consultant (IBCLC) in the United States through leadership, advocacy, professional development, and research.

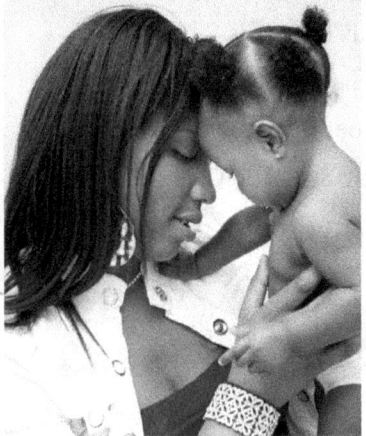

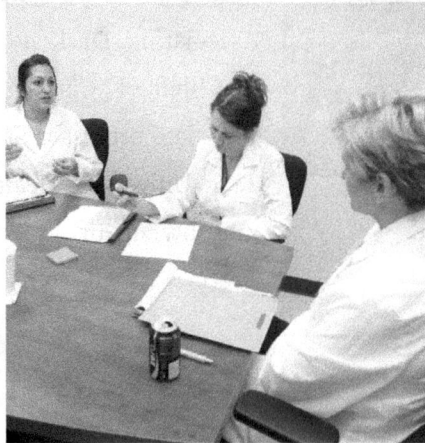

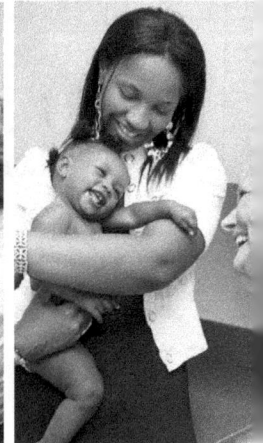

The U.S. Lactation Consultant Association Presents
Clinical Lactation Monographs

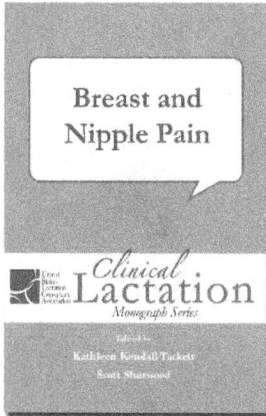

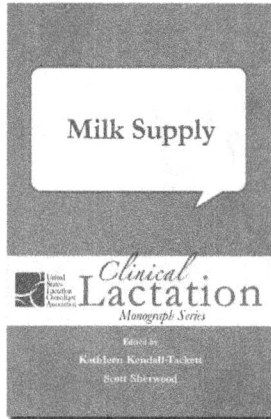

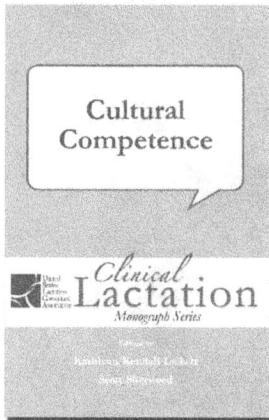

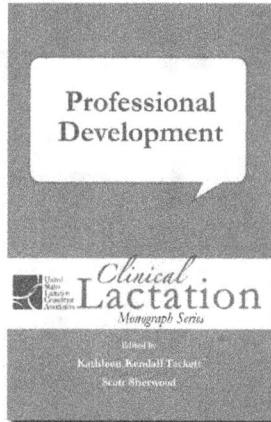

Praeclarus Press
Excellence in Women's Health

www.PraeclarusPress.com

Breastfeeding Titles from Praeclarus Press

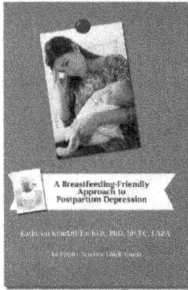

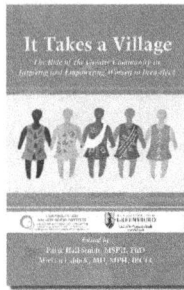

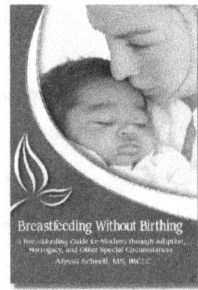

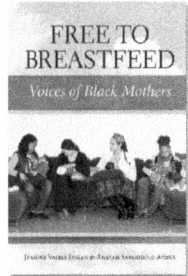

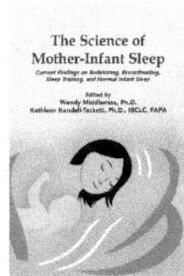

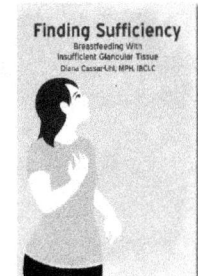

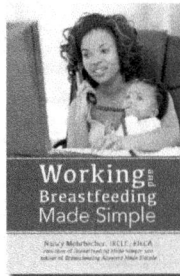

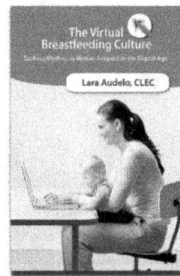

A Breastfeeding-Friendly Approach to Postpartum Depression

It Takes a Village

Breastfeeding Without Birthing

FREE TO BREASTFEED
Voices of Black Mothers

The Science of Mother-Infant Sleep

Finding Sufficiency
Breastfeeding With Insufficient Glandular Tissue

Working & Breastfeeding Made Simple

The Virtual Breastfeeding Culture
Lara Audelo, CLEC

Praeclarus Press
Excellence in Women's Health

www.PraeclarusPress.com

www.ingramcontent.com/pod-product-compliance
Lightning Source LLC
Chambersburg PA
CBHW070902280326
41934CB00008B/1544